Victor Fernando Couto
Valéria A. P Di Lorenzo
Alessandro dos S. Pin

Combined physical training for elderly patients with COPD

Victor Fernando Couto
Valéria A. P Di Lorenzo
Alessandro dos S. Pin

Combined physical training for elderly patients with COPD

Aerobic and resistance training in changing pneumological and muscular indicators

Imprint

Any brand names and product names mentioned in this book are subject to trademark, brand or patent protection and are trademarks or registered trademarks of their respective holders. The use of brand names, product names, common names, trade names, product descriptions etc. even without a particular marking in this work is in no way to be construed to mean that such names may be regarded as unrestricted in respect of trademark and brand protection legislation and could thus be used by anyone.

Cover image: www.ingimage.com

This book is a translation from the original published under ISBN 978-613-9-62115-6.

Publisher:
Sciencia Scripts
is a trademark of
Dodo Books Indian Ocean Ltd. and OmniScriptum S.R.L publishing group

120 High Road, East Finchley, London, N2 9ED, United Kingdom
Str. Armeneasca 28/1, office 1, Chisinau MD-2012, Republic of Moldova, Europe
Printed at: see last page
ISBN: 978-620-7-71332-5

SUMMARY

ACKNOWLEDGMENTS

First of all to **God**, because without him this study would not have been possible.

To my parents, **Valdette Regina Gardelin Couto and Paulo Fernando Couto**, for their encouragement and patience during difficult times.

To my great friends, **Gualberto Ruas** and **Maria Aparecida Borges Ruas,** who have always been with me, especially in times of difficulty, my eternal thanks.

To the entire research team at the Special Unit of Respiratory Physiotherapy (UEFR), especially those who contributed directly to the execution of this study: **Glaucia Nency Takara, Cilso Dias Paes, Bruna Varanda Pessoa and Ivana Gonçalves Labadessa.**

To my advisor, **Prof. Dr. Valéria Amorim Pires Di Lorenzo**, for the shared knowledge that certainly contributed to the conclusion of this important stage of my academic training, for her patience and for all the moments (good and bad) that provided me with rich learning about life.

To **Prof. Dr. Mauricio Jamami,** for making available the equipment and structure of the UEFR and, of course, for his patience and for the moments that provided me with rich learning experiences.

To the pulmonologists, **Dr. Fernando Tedesco and Dr. Antônio Delfino de Oliveira Junior**, for referring the COPD patients included in this study.

To the **patients and volunteers** for their cooperation, patience, friendship and learning.

To the examining board, Prof. **Dr. Fabio de Oliveira Pitta, Prof.ª . Dr. Audrey Borghi Silva and Prof. Dr. Victor Dourado**, for all the criticisms and suggestions that enriched this work.

The secretary of the Postgraduate Program in Physiotherapy (PPGFT), **Kelly Legoro**, for always being willing to help and for all the information that contributed to making the bureaucratic aspects easier to resolve.

INTRODUCTION:

Combined physical training (CPT) has been shown to be beneficial in improving exercise tolerance in elderly individuals with and without COPD. However, there is little evidence showing its impact on isolated prognostic indices and on the reduction in the BODE index in elderly people with COPD. **Objectives: To** compare the impact of a combination of aerobic and resistance training of the lower limbs on exercise tolerance, body composition and peripheral muscle strength in elderly individuals with and without COPD, as well as to evaluate the impact of this training on the BODE index in elderly individuals with COPD. **Methods:** This study included 18 male subjects, nine of whom were elderly people with COPD (GDPOC) and nine apparently healthy elderly people (GS). All subjects were assessed for lung function, distance covered in the six-minute walk test, cycle ergometer incremental test (CIT), cycle ergometer endurance test (TEC), body composition variables and 1-repetition maximum (1RM) leg press test. In addition to these variables, the GDPOC individuals were assessed for dyspnea and total score on the BODE index. The training consisted of thirty minutes of aerobic training at 60-70% of the incremental test on the cycle ergometer (TIC) and then three sets of fifteen repetitions of resistance training of the lower limbs on the leg press at an intensity of 40-60% of the 1RM test. Between the end of the aerobic training and the start of the resistance training, the individuals underwent five minutes of recovery. **Results:** After the CBT period, a significant difference was observed in the distance covered in the 6MWT in both the GDPOC and GS subjects. In the GDPOC, after the CBT, there was a significant increase in the peak load (Wpeak) of the CIT; in the time limit (T. Lim) of the CIT; in the load of the 1RM test, and a significant reduction in the total score of the BODE index.

CONCLUSION:

Combined physical training improved exercise tolerance, as evidenced by the greater distance covered in the 6MWT in both elderly individuals with and without COPD. We also observed that the CBT program benefited the GDPOC more, as it led to an increase in Wpeak in the TIC, in T. lim in the TEC, in the maximum load supported in the 1RM test and a clinically significant reduction in the BODE index in elderly individuals with COPD, indicating a better prognosis.

Key words: COPD; elderly; physical training; exercise tolerance.

CONTEXT

Individuals with Chronic Obstructive Pulmonary Disease (COPD) are characterized by chronic airflow obstruction that is not completely reversible. This obstruction is progressive and is related to the abnormal inflammatory response of the lungs to the inhalation of toxic gases, especially cigarette smoke[1].

Although this disease affects the lungs, there is various evidence of systemic inflammation, such as the presence of oxidative stress, high concentrations of circulating cytokines and activation of inflammatory cells, contributing to the development of hypermetabolism and a reduction in body mass index, which is an important factor in hospitalization[2,3].

Another alteration occurs as a result of chronic sedentary lifestyle, which leads to altered muscle phosphocreatine metabolism, increased muscle fatigue, resulting in reduced functional capacity[4]. This, in turn, reduces peripheral muscle strength, resulting in an even more intense ventilatory demand for the same dynamic activities, closing a cycle called dyspnea - sedentary lifestyle - dyspnea[4]. In addition, they cause a significant reduction in the cross-sectional area of the peripheral muscles of the lower limbs[5], compared to healthy individuals.

Muscle loss in the lower limbs, also seen in these individuals, leads to functional limitations, reducing their capacity for physical effort and compromising their performance in activities of daily living[6].

For this reason and due to the severity of the disease[4], they carried out a multicenter study to evaluate the factors that should determine the mortality of these individuals and developed the BODE *index (Body mass index; airflow Obstruction; Dyspnea and Exercise capacity)* index, which includes nutritional status by body mass index (BMI), airflow limitation verified by forced expiratory volume in the first second (FEV1), dyspnea sensation by the *Medical Research Council* (MRC) scale and exercise capacity by the six-minute walk test (6MWT).

In addition to the systemic changes caused by COPD itself and the fact that this disease affects elderly individuals, it is important to consider that with ageing there is a natural process of decline in the strength of skeletal muscles, respiratory muscles and body mass index (BMI), interfering with functional capacity and leading to exercise intolerance; and when these elderly people develop COPD, functional losses are accentuated due to the systemic manifestations caused by this disease[7,8,9] .

FUNCTIONAL ASSESSMENT TESTS

Functional assessment tests aim to evaluate functional capacity, effort tolerance, limitations to physical effort, responses to interventions[10,11] , reflecting an important component in predicting mortality and morbidities .[12,13]

One of the most widely used functional tests is the six-minute walk test (6MWT) because it is an easy, safe, low-cost, non-invasive test that is well accepted by elderly individuals[14,15] . In addition, the 6MWT is considered a good marker of functional capacity in ADLs[10,11] and the effort required in this test reflects the effort of individuals with COPD during ADLs, in addition to the reduction in distance covered reproducing the limitations of this population .[13]

On the other hand, the cycle ergometer incremental test (CIT) aims to subject the patient to programmed and personalized physical stress in order to evaluate the clinical, hemodynamic and electrocardiographic response. This evaluation makes it possible to detect stress-induced hemodynamic disorders, assess functional capacity, prescribe exercise and objectively evaluate the results of therapeutic interventions[14] .

The cycle ergometer endurance test (TEC) aims to assess respiratory capacity and tolerance to exertion. These assessments are made by measuring the time limit that the individual can tolerate in this test.

Based on the assessment of functional capacity through these tests, it is possible to direct an individualized intervention, taking into account all the changes described that lead to an intolerance to physical exercise, with physical and aerobic training being considered an important therapeutic strategy, acting to reverse the deconditioning resulting from the inactivity present in most of these individuals with COPD, providing an increase in the capacity for effort, strength and endurance of the peripheral muscles, improving tolerance to physical exercise and quality of life.

COMBINED PHYSICAL TRAINING (CPHT)

Lower limb aerobic training consistently results in an increase in endurance in individuals with COPD. However, this training has little effect on peripheral muscle weakness and atrophy, which are common problems reported by these individuals and contribute to exercise intolerance[15,16] .

The combination of aerobic and resistance exercise training has been shown to improve exercise tolerance, strength and peripheral muscle endurance of the lower limbs in apparently healthy elderly individuals and those affected by chronic respiratory diseases such as COPD[17,18] .

The combination of resistance and aerobic training over a 12-week period resulted in an increase in peripheral muscle mass and exercise tolerance compared to individuals who only performed aerobic training[19,20] .

The length of the training program has been much discussed, but still without consensual scientific support. From the available data, the literature assumes that longer training programs produce more benefits in terms of physiological adaptations[21,22] . However, there have been improvements in physical performance in terms of resistance to fatigue with an increase in the distance covered in the 6-minute walk test and in health status in programs of 6 to 12 weeks . [23,24,25,26.]

As a result, elderly individuals with COPD showed a reduction in the prognosis of the disease[5] , measured by the BODE index (*B - body mass index; O - airflow obstruction; D - dyspnea; E - exercise capacity*), which not only assesses the degree of obstruction of the disease, but also factors such as exercise tolerance and body mass index.

Although the combination of aerobic and resistance exercise training has been shown to be beneficial in improving exercise tolerance in individuals with COPD, there is still not enough scientific evidence to prove its impact on body composition, exercise tolerance and the predictive indices that assess the prognosis of the disease, which is why this study was carried out.

BIBLIOGRAPHICAL REFERENCES

1. Brazilian Society of Pulmonology and Phthisiology. II Brazilian Consensus on Tuberculosis: Brazilian Guidelines for Tuberculosis 2004. J Bras Pneumol. 2004; 30:S1-S42.

2. Godoy, I, Donahoe, M, Calhoun, WJ, Mancino, J, Rogers, RM. Elevated TNF-alpha production by peripheral blood monocytes of weight-losing COPD patients. Am J Respir Crit Care Med. 1996;153:633-637.

3. Prescott, E, Almdal, T, Mikkelsem, KL, Tofteng, CL, Vestbo, J, Lange, P. Prognostic value of weight change in chronic obstructive pulmonary disease: results from the Copenhagen City Heart Study. Eur Respir J. 2002; 20:539-544.

4. Celli, RB, Cote, GC, Marin, MJ, Pinto-Prata, V, Cabral, JH. The Body-Mass, airflow obstruction, dyspnea, and exercise capacity index in chronic obstructive pulmonary disease. N Engl J Med. 2004; 350:1005-12.

5. Whitton, F, Jobin, J, Simard, PM, Lebranc, P, Simard, C, Bernard, S. Histochemical and morphological characteristics of the vastus lateralis muscle in patients with chronic obstructive pulmonary disease. Med Sci Sports Exerc. 1998; 30:1467-1474.

6. Yoshikawa, M, Yoneda, T, Takenaka, H, Fukuoka, A, Okamoto, Y, Narita, N, Nezu, K. Distribution of muscle mass and maximal exercise performance in patients with COPD. Chest. 2001; 11:93-8.

7. Summerhill, EM, Angov, N, Garber, C, Mccol, FD. Respiratory muscle strength in the physically active elderly. Lung. 2007; 185:315-20.

8. Dourado, VZ, Tanni, SE, Vale, AS, Faganello, MM, Godoy, I. Systemic manifestations in chronic obstructive pulmonary disease. J Bras. Pneumol. 2006; 32:161-71.

9. Doherty, TJ. Invited review: Aging and sarcopenia. J Appl Physiol. 2003; 95:171727.

10. Leung, ASY, Chan, KK, Sykes, K, Chan, KS. Reliability, validity and responsiveness of two minutes walk test to assess exercise capacity of COPD patients. Chest. 2006; 130:119-25.

11. Casas, A, Vilaro, J, Rabinovich, R, Mayer, A, Barbera, JÂ, Rodrigues-Roisin, R. Encouraged 6 min walking test indicates maximun sustainable exercise in COPD patients. Chest. 2005; 128:55-61.

12. Neder, JA, Nery, LE. Clinical Exercise Physiology: Theory and Practice. Editora Artes Médicas. 2003.

13. Wegner, RE, Jorres, RA, Kirsten, DK, Magnussen, H. Factor analysis of exercise capacity, dyspnea ratings and lung function in patients with severe COPD. Eur Respir J. 1994; 7:725-9.

14. ATS Statement: Guidelines for the six minute walk tests. ATS Committee on Proficiency Standards for Clinical Pulmonary Function Laboratories. Am J Respir Crit Care Med. 2002; 166:111-7.

15. Solway, S. A qualitative systematic overview of the measurement properties of functional walk test used in the cardiorespiratory domain. Chest. 2001; 119:256-270.

16. Brazilian Society of Cardiology. Guidelines on Exercise Testing. Arq Bras Cardiol. 2002; 78:2.

17. Mador, MJ, Bozkanet, E, Aggarwal, A, Shaffer, M, Kuffer, TJ. Endurance and strength training in patients with COPD. Chest. 2001; 125:2036-45.

18. Casaburi, R. Skeletal muscle function in COPD. Chest. 2000; 117.

19. Silva, TA, Frisioli, JA, Pinheiro, MM, Szejnfeld, VL. Sarcopenia associated with aging: etiological aspects and therapeutic options. Rev Bras Reumatol. 2006; 46(6):391-7.

20. Nelson, ME, Rejeski, WJ, Blair, SN, Duncan, PW, Judge, JO, King, AC. Physical activity and public health in older adults: recommendat ion from the American College of Sports Medicine and the American Heart Association. Med Sci Sports Exerc. 2007; 39:1435-45.

21. Bernard, S, Whitton, F, Lebranc, P, Jobin, J, Belleau, R, Carrier, G, Maltais, F. Aerobic and strength training in patients with chronic obstructive pulmonary disease. Am J Respir Crit Care Med. 1999; 159:896-901.

22. Sala, E, Roca, J, Marrades, RM, Alonso, J, Gonzalez, JM, Moreno, A. Effects of endurance training on skeletal muscle bioenergetics in chronic obstructive pulmonary disease. Am J Respir Crit Care Med. 1999; 159:1726 -1734.

23. Puente-Maestu, L, Santacruz, A, Vargas, T, Martinez, Y, Whipp, BJ. Effects of training on the tolerance to high -intensity exercise in patients with severe COPD. Respiration. 2003; 70:367 -370.

24. Troosters, T, Gosselink, R, Decramer, M. Short and long -term effects of outpatient rehabilitation in patients with chronic obstructive pulmonary disease: a randomized trial. Am J Med. 2000; 109:207 -212.

25. Green, RH, Singh, SJ, Williams, J, Morgan, MDL. A randomized controlled trial of four weeks versus seven weeks of pulmonary rehabilitation in chronic obstructive pulmonary disease. Thorax. 2001; 56:143 -145.

26. Ortega, F, Toral, J, Cejudo, P, Villagomez, R, Sanchez, H, Castillo, J. Comparison of effects of strength and endurance training in patients with chronic obstructive pulmonary disease. Am J Respir Crit Care Med. 2002, 166:669 -674.

27. Mckeough, ZJ, Alison, JA, Bye, PT, Trenell, MI, Sachinwalla, T, Thompson, CH. Exercise capacity and quadriceps muscle metabolism following training in

subjects with COPD. Respir Med. 2006; 100:1817-1825.

28. Spruit, MA, Gosselink, R, Troosters, T, De Paepe, K, Decramer, M. Resistance versus endurance training in patients with COPD and peripheral muscle weakness. Eur Respir J. 2002; 19:1072-1078.

INTRODUCTION

The combination of aerobic and resistance training has been shown to be beneficial in improving exercise tolerance, strength, lower limb peripheral muscle endurance, as well as being more tolerable in healthy elderly individuals and those affected by chronic respiratory diseases such as Chronic Obstructive Pulmonary Disease (COPD)[1,2] . This training has two different types: long-duration, in which strength training is added to the existing aerobic training, increasing the duration of the sessions[3,4] and short-duration, in which the duration of the aerobic training session is halved and the other half of the session is dedicated to strength training .[5,6]

It is important to consider that with ageing there is a natural process of decline in the strength of skeletal muscles, respiratory muscles and body mass index (BMI) interfering with functional capacity, leading to exercise intolerance; and when these elderly develop COPD, functional losses are accentuated due to the systemic manifestations that this disease entails[7-9] .

The systemic manifestations related to this disease, such as the increase in the inflammatory process due to the higher concentration of circulating cytokines, and oxidative stress, lead to the development of hypermetabolism[10] , contributing to weight loss, associated with a reduction in lean body mass, which results in peripheral skeletal muscle dysfunction, predominantly in the lower limbs, compromising the ability to perform physical exercise[11] . These manifestations lead to an increase in ventilatory demand, a feeling of dyspnea, contributing to limitations in activities of daily living (ADLs)[11] and, above all, compromising the quality of life of these individuals, who may present recurrent exacerbations as the disease progresses, constituting an important risk factor for hospitalization, as well as indicating a worse prognosis in the evolution of the exacerbation and survival of these patients[8] .

With these manifestations in mind, a multidimensional index and predictor of COPD prognosis was created, called the BODE index[11] . This index is made up of four variables (*B - body mass index; O - airflow obstruction; D - dyspnea; E - exercise capacity*), of which three (*B - body mass index; D - dyspnea; E - exercise capacity*) can be modified by physical training.

In the study by Bernard et al (1999), the combination of resistance and aerobic training lasting 12 weeks resulted in an increase in peripheral muscle mass and exercise tolerance compared to individuals who only performed aerobic training.

Combined physical training lasting 12 weeks has been identified as the best strategy[12,13] , as it shows a 15% increase in the number of capillaries per fiber and a 38% increase in the activity of citrate synthase, an important enzyme involved in oxidative metabolism[13,5,14,6] .

There have been few studies describing the impact of a combination of aerobic and resistance training of the lower limbs on exercise tolerance and body mass index in elderly people with and without COPD, as well as the benefits of short-term combined training on the BODE index in elderly people with COPD, justifying this study.

Thus, we hypothesize that short-term combined physical training is capable of providing adaptations in body composition, exercise tolerance and reducing the total score of the BODE index in individuals with COPD.

OBJECTIVE

To compare the impact of aerobic and resistance training of the lower limbs on exercise tolerance as assessed by the endurance test on the cycle ergometer (TEC) and the distance covered in the six-minute walk test, peripheral muscle strength and body composition among elderly individuals with and without a lower limb.

COPD and evaluate the impact of this training on the BODE index in elderly individuals with COPD.

Inclusion and Exclusion Criteria

This study included apparently healthy elderly individuals with COPD who had been clinically stable for four weeks prior to the evaluations, aged between 60 and 80 years, male, non-smokers, with no neurological, rheumatic or orthopedic problems, or recent lower limb surgeries that could prevent them from performing the tests.

Individuals with uncontrolled systemic arterial hypertension, peripheral oxygen saturation (Sp_{O2}) below 88% at rest and who did not agree to sign the consent form were excluded.

casuistry and methods

We assessed 14 individuals with COPD who had been referred to the special respiratory physiotherapy laboratory (LEFIR) at UFSCar by pulmonologists in the city of Sao Carlos. Of these, 11 completed the assessments; however, two were excluded during the physical training sessions, one due to a respiratory exacerbation and the other due to withdrawal. Thus, 9 males completed all the stages of this study and made up the COPD group (GDPOC).

This group consisted of one individual with mild obstruction, three with moderate obstruction, four with severe obstruction and one with very severe obstruction according to the GOLD criteria, 2008.

The group of apparently healthy individuals (SG) was made up of 9 males recruited from the Open University for the Third Age in the city of Sao Carlos.

All the individuals agreed to take part in this study, signing a free and informed consent form in accordance with Resolution 196/96 of the National Health Council (CNS), which was approved by the UFSCar Research Ethics Committee (Opinion No. 272/2010).

Elderly individuals with and without COPD were assessed and re-evaluated after six weeks of short-term combined lower limb exercise training in terms of body composition, pulmonary function, peripheral muscle strength, endurance and distance covered, which was measured using the six-minute walk test. The Medical Research Council (MRC) scale and the BODE index total score were only applied to the GDPOC.

EXPERIMENTAL PROCEDURE

1) Lung Function Assessment

Pulmonary function was assessed using a properly calibrated spirometer (microQuark PC-based spirometer Cosmed®), following the Guidelines of the Brazilian Society of Pulmonology and Phthisiology (2002), and FEV1 values were obtained to classify the severity and prognosis of COPD before and after the physical training program, using the BODE index.

The values obtained were compared with those predicted by Pereira (2007), according to age, height, gender, race and weight.

2) Body Composition Assessment

Body composition was assessed and reassessed using a bioelectrical impedance scale (*Tanita*® *, model BC-553*). For this purpose, all the individuals fasted for at least 4 hours in order to standardize their liquid intake.

They were instructed to wear light clothing, to drink water and to remove all objects to avoid altering the values obtained on the scales.

This assessment was carried out with the individuals in the orthostatic position, enabling analysis of weight, % body fat (%BF), % muscle mass (%MM) and body mass index (BMI)[16-18] .

3)   Medical Research Council (MRC) Scale

The MRC scale was applied during the assessment and reassessment of elderly individuals with COPD in order to assess the extent to which dyspnea limits their activities of daily living (ADLs). These individuals reported their subjective degree of dyspnea by choosing a value between 0 and 4[19] .

4)   Six Minute Walk Test (6MWT)

The 6MWT was carried out in a flat corridor 30 meters long and 1.5 meters wide. All the individuals were instructed and encouraged to walk as fast as possible for six minutes, using standardized phrases every minute. After the six minutes were up, the distance covered was measured[20] .

During the test, SpO2 values (*Nonin*[®] , 2500), heart rate (HR) (*Polar*® model T31) were observed along with the application of the Borg CR 10 scale (EB-CRlO) to assess the sensation of dyspnea and lower limb fatigue every minute[20] .

If the individual had an intense feeling of dyspnea, lower limb fatigue, SpO_2 below 85% and/or reached submaximal heart rate, they were allowed to rest in the orthostatic position, with the stopwatch on, and instructed to continue the test as soon as they had $SpO_2 \geq 90\%$, submaximal HR below the predicted value and EB- CR10 $\leq$ 3 until the end of the sixth minute. After carrying out this test, we calculated the expected distance covered for the Brazilian population[21] .

5) BODE index

The BODE index was used to assess the prognosis of elderly individuals with COPD before and after six weeks of physical training.

The four variables that make it up were considered (0-3 for VEFi, MRC scale and distance walked in the 6MWT, while BMI values of 0-1 will be obtained)[11] in isolation and also the total score for these individuals, as shown in table i.

Table 1 - BODE index total score

Variables	0	1	2	3
VEFi (% prev)	$\geq$65	50-64	36-49	$\leq$35
SD of the 6MWT	$\geq$350	250-349	150-249	$\leq$149
MRC scale	0-1	2	3	4
BMI (kg/m)^2	$\geq$21	$\leq$21		

FEV1 = Forced expiratory volume in the first second; SD = distance walked; 6MWT = six-minute walk test; MRC scale = Medical Research Council scale; BMI = body mass index.

6) Cycle ergometer incremental test (TIC)

The intensity for aerobic training was determined by the symptom-limiting incremental test using the modified BALKE protocol[22] , which is an incremental protocol of increasing load and constant speed.

In this test, each individual warmed up for 3 minutes on a stationary bike (*Ergo 167 Cycle*), using a minimum load of 15 watts.

Subsequently, 10 watts were increased every 2 minutes, at the end of which SpO2 values were collected (*Nonin*® 2500), HR using a frequency meter (*polar*® model T31), blood pressure (BP) (*Diasyst*®) and sensation of dyspnea and fatigue in the lower limbs (EB-CR10). In addition, all the subjects' heart rate was monitored using an electrocardiograph (*Medtec*® model *Ecafix*).

The test was stopped when the individual showed signs and symptoms in accordance with the Brazilian Society of Cardiology Guidelines on Exercise Testing[23] .

7)   Cycle ergometer endurance test (TEC)

This test was carried out on a bicycle ergometer (Ergo 167 Cycle), to observe each individual's time limit, using a constant load of 70% of the TIC (modified BALKE)[25] .

SpO2 (*Nonin*[®] 2500), HR (*polar*[®] model T31), BP (*Diasyst®*) and sensation of dyspnea and lower limb fatigue (EB-CR10) were collected while the individual was at rest on the bike. During the test, these variables were collected every two minutes until the individual became intolerant.

The test was stopped if the individual showed signs and symptoms in accordance with the II Brazilian Society of Cardiology Guidelines on Exercise Testing, 2002.

8)   1 Repetition Maximum Test (1RM)

This test consists of determining the greatest amount of weight that the individual can move once, on a horizontal leg press (*Righetto PR1070*), while the initial load for the test was 60% of the body weight[24] , and if they managed to complete a repetition or not, the amount of weight used was increased or reduced respectively, and 1RM was performed again, with a minimum interval of two minutes between each load used. Each individual had a limit of six attempts to obtain the load[25] . If they were unable to determine the load within 6 attempts, they performed the test again after 48 hours, thus avoiding a possible overload on the cardiovascular system and skeletal muscle damage. It should also be noted that on the first day of the evaluation, the individual adapted to the equipment (*Righetto PR1070*), thus eliminating the learning effect.

9)   Short-term Combined Physical Training

This program was carried out over a period of six weeks, three times a week, consisting of aerobic and resistance training of the lower limbs.

The aerobic training of each individual was carried out on a stationary bike (*Ergo 167 Cycle*) for 30 minutes maintaining a load of 60% of the TIC, with a 10% increase after three weeks of training[5,26,27,28] .

During this session, BP (*Diasyst®*), SpO_2 (*Nonin®* 2500), HR *(polar®* model T31) and feelings of dyspnea and lower limb fatigue (EB- CR10) were observed every two minutes. If the individual had dyspnea and/or lower limb fatigue > 5, SpO_2 equal to or less than 85%, HR above the submaximal value, a two-minute break was taken and the individual remained seated on the bicycle, where they returned once the physical variables had normalized ($SpO_2 \geq 90\%$, submaximal HR below the predicted value and EB-CR10 ≤ 3)[23] .

After the end of this training session, the individuals underwent five minutes of recovery to normalize the physical variables.

Resistance training for the lower limbs consisted of three sets of fifteen repetitions[29,30] on a horizontal leg press (*Righetto PR1070*), where the subjects rested for two minutes at the end of each set.

The intensity of this training was between 40-60% of the maximum load tolerated in the 1 repetition maximum (1RM) test, with a 10% increase every two weeks.

Figure 1: Sample design of the short ldura çà o combined physical training program.

Figura 1: Desenho amostral do programa de treinamento físico combinado de curta duração.

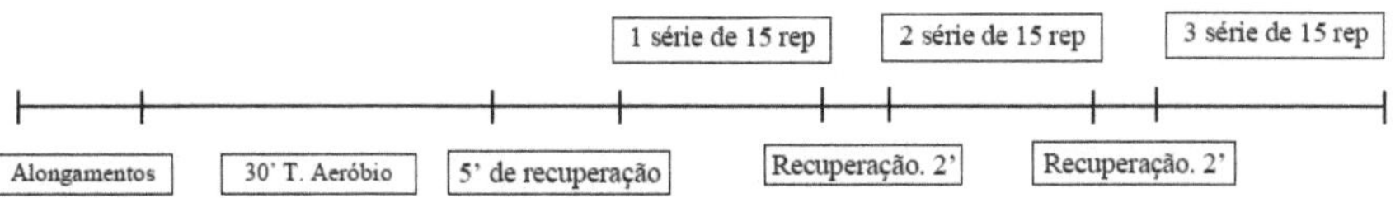

Statistical Analysis

The *Shapiro Wilk* test was used to check the distribution of the data.

The data were expressed as medians and interquartile ranges as they are non-parametric.

For intra-group analysis, the *Wilcoxon* test was used, while for inter-group analysis the unpaired T-test was used for parametric data and the *Mann-Whitney test* for non-parametric data.

The statistical program used was the Statistical Package for the Social Sciences (SPSS) version 13.0 for Windows. The significance level was p<0.05.

To calculate the sample power, the standard deviation and difference in means were used to obtain a minimum clinically significant difference of a reduction of 1.0 point in the BODE index, which resulted in a sample size of 15 individuals.

RESULTS

Of the individuals included in the GDPOC, two had co-morbidities in addition to respiratory disease, one with osteophytes at the T2 and T7 levels of the spine, while the other had asymptomatic arthrosis of the left knee. As for the healthy individuals, none had co-morbidities.

With regard to the body mass index (BMI) of the individuals with COPD included in this study, we found that two were undernourished (BMI <20 kg/m^2), four had a normal BMI (BMI: 20 - 24.9 kg/m^2) and three were overweight (BMI: 25 - 29.9 kg/m).^{2}

For the apparently healthy individuals, we found that five had a normal BMI (BMI: 20 - 24.9 kg/m^2) and four were overweight (BMI: 25 - 29.9 kg/m^2) (PRESCOTT et al, 2002).

The anthropometric, spirometric and body composition characteristics of the COPD (GDPOC) and apparently healthy (GS) individuals included in this study are described in Table 2. There were no differences in age, weight and height between the GDPOC and GS individuals. The spirometric variables of the GDPOC were significantly lower than those of the GS, characterizing airway obstruction.

There were no significant differences in body composition before and after six weeks of short-term combined training.

In relation to physical exercise, the distance covered in the 6MWT was significantly lower in the GDPOC when compared to the SG. Both groups showed a significant increase in PD after CBT (table 3).

Table 3 also shows the median total score of the BODE index and its variables, where there is a significant difference between the groups in the variables, body mass index (BMI) and distance covered in the six-minute walk test.

After the period of short-term combined physical training, the total score of the BODE index decreased significantly from pre- to post-training (3 (2.1-4) vs. 2 (1.4-3)) in the GDPOC subjects (table 3).

In Table 4, the muscle strength variable assessed by the 1RM test also showed a significant difference after this physical training, being significantly higher in the GDPOC.

The TIC and TEC performance of the GDPOC and GS individuals before and after six weeks of short-term combined physical training is also shown in Table 4.

In the GDPOC, two individuals stopped the TIC during the evaluation period because they reached submaximal HR. After the six-week training period, only one individual stopped this test. As for the GS, no individual stopped the test.

Table 1 - Characteristics of the sample of individuals studied.

Variables	GDPOC (n=9)	GS (n=9)
	Median (Interquartile)	**Median (Interquartile)**
Sex	9 men	9 men
Age	71 (68-75,3)	66 (59,8-70,7)
Height (cm)	167 (163,7-170,3)	175 (168,7-177,9)
Weight (Kg)	71 (61,8-78,1)	72 (65,4-85,9)
BMI (kg/m$)^2$	24,5 (21,6-26,9)	24,9 (21,7-27,9)
FEV1% (L)	46,6 (37,3-64)	108,6 (97,8-116,9)*
FEV1 (L)	1,25 (0,9-1,7)	3,36 (3,1-3,7)*
FVC (%)	71,4 (61,4-74)	116,6 (106,8-127,2)*
FVC (L)	2,1 (1,6-2,5)	4,28 (3,9-5,1)*
FEV1/FVC %	65,2 (56,4-72,8)	96,2 (88,8-99,6)*
GC (%)	27 (22,4-31,6)	22,3 (18,9-32,3)
MM (%)	49 (43,3-51,9)	51,2 (48,3-55,7)
SD (% prev)	88,2	99,2
SD (m)	486 (371-530,7)	560 (493,8-646,2)*
Baseline SpO2 (%)	93 (92-95)	97 (95-98)
BODE (total score) 3 (2.1-4.1)		-

BMI= Body Mass Index; FEV1= Forced Expiratory Volume in the first second; FVC= Forced Vital Capacity; MI= Percentage of Metabolic Age; MO= Percentage of Bone Mass; GC= Percentage of Body Fat; MM= Percentage of Lean Mass; SD= Distance Walked; SpO2= Peripheral Oxygen Saturation; BODE= Body Mass Index, Airway Obstruction, Dyspnea and Exercise Capacity Index. *Statistically significant difference (unpaired t-test) ($p < 0.05$) between groups.

Table 3 - Impact of short-term CBT on body composition components, total BODE score and its variables.

Variables GDPOC (n=9)		GS (n=9)	
Median (Interquartile)		**Median (Interquartile)**	
Pre	Post	Pre	Post

Weight	71 (61,8-78,1)	71,2 (62-79,1)	71,5 (64,2-85)	73 (64,8-84,7)
GC (%)	27 (22.4-31.6)	25.8 (22.4-32)	22,3 (19-32,3)	22,7 (18,6-31,4)
MM (%)	49 (43.4-51.8)	51 (44.7-52.6)	51,2 (48,3-55,3)	51,3 (48,4-56,3)
IMC (%)	24,6(21,6-26, 27,7)*	9)26,2(22,8-	24,9 (21,7-27,8)	25 (21,8-27,7)£
			108,2 (101-112,4)	108,6 (102-114)
VEF1 % (L)	46.6 (37.3-63.9)	47.5 (39.1-67.3)	--	
MRC1	,3 (0,5-1,2)	1 (0,6-1,1)	560 (493-646)	642 (541-684)*£
SD (m)	486 (371-530)	558 (457-606)*	82 (74-84)	--
Δ DP (m)		72 (65-78)		
BODE3 index	(2.1-4)	2 (1.4-3)*		

GC= Body Fat Percentage; MM= Lean Mass Percentage; BMI= Body Mass Index; FEV1= Forced Expiratory Volume in the first second; MRC= Medical Research Council Scale; SD= Distance walked in the 6MWT; Δ SD= Delta gain in distance walked after short-term CBT; BODE= Body Mass Index, Airway Obstruction, Dyspnea and exercise capacity. *Statistically significant (p < 0.05) intra-group difference (*Wilcoxon* test)

£ Statistically significant difference (unpaired t-test) (p < 0.05) between groups.

Table 4 - Effects of short-term CBT on Wpeak in the TIC; T. threshold in the TEC; distance covered; feeling of dyspnea and fatigue in the lower limbs in the 6MWT and 1RM test.

Variables	GDPOC		GS	
	Median (Interquartile)		Median (Interquartile)	
	Pre	Post	Pre	Post
Wpeak (watts)	30 (26.6-42.2)	40 (30,7-47)*	60 (42,5-67,5)	65 (49,2-73)
T. lim TE (min)	9 (7-16.3)	31 (14,7-30,8)*	31 (19-32,7)	31 (22,8-33)
DP (m)	486 (371-530)	558 (457-606)*	560 (493-646)	642 (541-684)*£
Dyspnea 2 min	1 (1.3-1.9)	1 (1,1-1,6)	0 (0,07-0,2)	0 (0,06-0,1)
Dyspnea 6 min	3 (1.9-2.6)	3 (2,0-2,5)	0 (0,1-0,4)	0 (0,2-0,3)
Lower limbs 2 min	1 (0.26-1.6)	0,5 (0,2-0,9)	0 (0,02-0,4)	0 (0-0,28)

| Lower limbs 6 min2 (0.8-3.1) | 1 (0,4-2,2) | 0,5 (0,01-1,6) | 0 (-0,26-1,2) |
| 1RM (Kg) 60 (49.9-70.5) | 80 (65,3-82,4)* | 80 (68,7-87,4) | 80 (70,5-88,3) |

Wpico= Peak load in the cycle ergometer incremental test; T. lim TE= Time limit in the cycle ergometer Endurance Test lim TE= Time limit in the Endurance Test on a cycle ergometer; SD= Distance covered; Dyspnea 2 min= Feeling of dyspnea during two minutes of the 6MWT; Dyspnea 6 min= Feeling of dyspnea during six minutes of the 6MWT; MMII 2 min= Feeling of tiredness in the MMII during two minutes of the 6MWT; MMII 6 min= Feeling of tiredness in the MMII during six minutes of the 6MWT; IRM= 1 Maximum Repetition Test;. *Statistically significant (p < 0.05) intra-group difference (*Wilcoxon* test).

DISCUSSION

In this study it was possible to observe that the combination of aerobic and resistance training of short duration is capable of generating a positive impact on exercise tolerance in elderly individuals with and without COPD. In addition, a significant improvement was observed in the BMI variable of body composition and a clinically relevant impact on the total score of the BODE index in individuals with COPD[31] .

Elderly individuals aged between 60 and 80 who were apparently healthy and had COPD took part in this study, with the aim of comparing functional losses with normal aging and gains with a lower limb CBT program.

Table 2 shows the anthropometric values, spirometry, body composition and distance covered in the 6MWT obtained during the evaluation period in these individuals. This table shows that there was a significant difference in spirometry values, which were lower in individuals with COPD compared to apparently healthy individuals. This result is due to airway obstruction, which is one of the factors that characterize COPD.

With regard to pre-training body composition, the lean mass (LM) variable showed lower values in individuals with COPD compared to apparently healthy individuals (49 (43.4-51.8) vs. 51.2 (48.3-55.3)) (table 3). This lower percentage of lean mass in these individuals has been attributed to atrophy due to disuse or physical deconditioning[8] . In studies[32,33] carried out on material collected from biopsies of the vastus lateralis muscle, it was observed that as a result of this deconditioning, individuals with COPD show a significant reduction in oxidative enzymes and/or an increase in glycolytic enzymes. Another bioenergetic alteration observed in these individuals was a reduction in muscle phosphocreatine metabolism, which is one of the main factors involved in anaerobic metabolism and leads to a greater feeling of tiredness and/or fatigue in the peripheral muscles. This in turn reduces strength and aerobic capacity, resulting in an even more intense ventilatory demand for dynamic activities[8] .

As a result of these changes, the GDPOC individuals who underwent short-term combined training for six weeks showed greater gains in MM compared to the GS individuals (Δ2 vs Δ0.1) (Table 3). As for the severity of the disease, individuals with severe and very severe COPD showed the greatest gains in MM (Δ3.7 %MM) compared to those with mild and moderate COPD. This shows that the greater the severity of the disease, the greater the benefits after physical training. However, it was not possible to analyze the data due to the insufficient number of elderly individuals with COPD with different degrees of obstruction.

The same was observed for the distance covered in the 6MWT, where the GDPOC individuals had shorter distances when compared to the SG individuals.

With regard to the gain in the distance covered in the six-minute walk test after the GDPOC intervention, it showed greater tolerance to physical exercise, as well as less feeling of fatigue in the lower limbs (2 (0.8-3.1) vs 1 (0.42.2)) in the 6MWT (Table 4).

In addition, in the distance traveled variable, individuals belonging to GDPOC and GS showed an increase of Δ72m vs Δ82m, respectively, and for individuals with COPD, a minimum difference of 35 m from baseline is considered a clinically important and significant factor[35] .

The six-minute walk test assessed cardiorespiratory capacity and is used in pulmonary rehabilitation programs to assess exercise tolerance, monitor the effectiveness of treatment and establish the prognosis of individuals with COPD[36] . The predicted values were obtained by averaging the results according to the formula by Iwama et al (2009). In this study, we found that elderly individuals with COPD had poor aerobic fitness, as they were below the predicted value (Table 2).

Based on the results of this study, the six-week period of short-term combined physical training had an impact on exercise tolerance in both apparently healthy elderly individuals and those with COPD, benefiting those with COPD more, due to the greater systemic and pulmonary involvement of these individuals as a result of the disease, as described above. The aerobic training intensity of 60-70% of TIC may have led to an increase in the concentration of capillaries, oxidative enzymes, mitochondrial density and a reduction in glycolytic enzymes, which are responsible for the feeling of fatigue in the lower limbs reported by elderly individuals with[DPOC] [8,37,4,38].

Although this intensity is considered low[5,14] , it showed an increase in the time limit of the ECT, an increase in the peak load (W) of the ECT and, as a consequence, an increase in the functional performance of the GDPOC individuals, as shown in this study.

The gain in strength of the lower limb muscles seen in the 1RM test (60 (49.9-70.5) vs 80 (65.3-82.4)) shows an improvement in peripheral muscular endurance, which is impaired in these individuals with COPD. The muscular endurance training carried out in this study used an intensity of 40-60% of the 1RM test, with the aim of gaining strength and endurance[29,14] . The combination of resistance training of the lower limbs can help improve exercise tolerance, since peripheral muscle limitation is one of the factors that leads to intolerance to physical exercise .[4]

In GDPOC individuals, we observed (Table 3) that after the six-week period of short-term combined physical training there was a significant increase in body mass index (24.6 (21.6-26.9) vs. 26,2 (22.8-27.7)), distance walked (486 (371-530) vs 558 (457-606)) and consequently a lower BODE total score (3 (2.1-4) vs 2 (1.4-3)), which is associated with COPD prognosis[31,34] .

In a study by Nasis et al, (2009), a one-point reduction in the BODE index was also observed after the same combined physical training. However, in order to present these results, these authors compared combined interval training with continuous combined training over a 12-week period, whereas in our study the same reduction was possible in just six weeks of training.

We therefore suggest that future studies should include interventions with low-intensity CBT and longer periods of time.

Limitations of the study

In this study, we consider that there were some limitations, such as the small number of individuals who made up both groups. Other limitations include the absence of a COPD control group and groups with different periods of CBT.

CONCLUSION

CBT improved exercise tolerance, as evidenced by the greater distance covered in the 6MWT in both elderly individuals with and without COPD. We also found that the CBT program benefited the GDPOC more, as it led to an increase in Wpeak in the TIC, in T. lim in the TEC, in the maximum load supported in the 1RM test and a clinically significant reduction in the BODE index in elderly individuals with COPD, indicating a better prognosis.

Bibliographical references

1. Silva, TA, Frisioli, JA, Pinheiro, MM, Szejnfeld, VL. Sarcopenia associated with aging: etiologic aspects and therapeutic options. Rev Bras Reumatol. 2006;46(6):391-7.

2. Nelson, ME, Rejeski, WJ, Blair, SN, Duncan, PW, Judge, JO, King, AC. Physical activity and public health in older adults: recommendation from the American College of Sports Medicine and the American Heart Association. Med Sci Sports Exerc. 2007;39:1435-45.

3. Dourado, VZ, Antunes, LCO, Tanni, SE, Gonçalves, RS, Rodrigues, H, Cavalcante, DM. Effects of different combinations of strength training and low intensity general reconditioning exercises in COPD patients. Eur Respir J. 2005;26.

4. Ortega, F, Toral, J, Cejudo, P, Villagomez, R, Sanchez, H, Castilho, J. Comparasion of effects of strength and endurance training in patients with chronic obstructive pulmonary disease. Am J Respir Crit Care Med. 2002;166:669-74.

5. Bernard, S, Whitton, F, Lebranc, P, Jobin, J, Belleau, R, Carrier, G, Maltais, F. Aerobic and strength training in patients with chronic obstructive pulmonary disease. Am J Respir Crit Care Med. 1999;159: 896-901.

6. Mador, MJ, Bozkanat, E, Aggarwal, A, Shaffer, M, Kuffer, TJ. Endurance and strength training in patients with COPD. Chest. 2004;125:2036-45.

7. Summerhill, EM, Angov, N, Garber, C, Mcool, FD. Respiratory muscle strength in the physically active elderly. Lung. 2007;185:315-20.

8. Dourado, VZ, Tanni, SE, Vale, AS, Faganello, MM, Godoy, I. Systemic manifestations in chronic obstructive pulmonary disease. J Bras. Pneumol. 2006;32:161-71.

9. Doherty, TJ. Invited review: Aging and sarcopenia. J Appl Physiol. 2003;95:1717-27.

10. Prescott, E, Almdal, T, Mikklsen, KL, Tofteng, CL, Vestbo, J, Lange, P. Prognostic value of weight change in chronic obstructive pulmonary disease: results from the Copenhagen City Heart Study. Eur Respir J. 2002;20:539-44.

11. Celli, RB, Cote, GC, Marin, MJ, Pinto-Prata, V, Cabral, JH. The Body-Mass, airflow obstruction, dyspnea, and exercise capacity index in chronic obstructive pulmonary disease. N Engl J Med. 2004;350:1005-12.

12. Hagerman, FC, Walsh, SJ, Staron, RS, Hikida, RS, Gilders, RM, Murray, TF, Toma, K, Ragg, KE. Effects of high-intensity resistance training on untrained older men. I. Stength, cardiovascular, and metabolic responses. J. Gerontol. Biol. Sci. Med. Sci. 2000;55:336-46.

13. Yoshikawa, M, Yoneda, T, Takenaka, H, Fukuoka, A, Okamoto, Y, Narita, N, Nezu, K. Distribution of muscle mass and maximal exercise performance in patients with COPD. Chest. 2001;11:93-8.

14. Panton, L, Golden, L, Broeder, CE, Browder, K, Seifer, FD. The effects of resistance training on functional outcomes in patients with chronic obstructive pulmonary disease. Eur J Appl Physiol. 2004;91:443-9.

15. Brazilian Society of Pulmonology and Phthisiology. Guidelines for pulmonary function tests. J Bras Pneumol. 2002;28(3).

16. Tribess, S, Petroski, L, Anez, CRR. Fat percentage in physical conditioning practitioners by bioelectrical impedance and anthropometric technique. Revista Digital. 2003;64.

17. Mendes, CCT, Raele, R. Body assessment by bioimpedance. Rev Nutr Pauta. 1997;24:12-4.

18. Rezende, A, Rosado, L, Franceschinni, S.; Rosado, G, Ribeiro, R, Marins, JCB. Critical review of available methods for assessing body composition in large population and clinical studies. Archivos Latinoamericanos de Nutricion. 2007;57.

19. Kovelis, D, Segretti, ON, Probst, VS, Lareau, SC, Brunetto, AB, Pitta, F. Validation of the Modified Pulmonary Functional Status and Dyspnea Questionnaire and the Medical Research Council scale for use in patients with chronic obstructive pulmonary disease in Brazil. J Bras Pneumol. 2008;34:1008-18.

20. ATS Statement: Guidelines for the six minute walk tests. ATS Committee on Proficiency Standards for Clinical Pulmonary Function Laboratories. Am J Respir Crit Care Med. 2002;166:111-7.

21. Iwama, AM, Andrade, GN, Shima, P, Tanni, SE, Godoy, I, Dourado, VZ. The six-minute walk test and body weight-walk distance product in healthy Brazilian subjects. Brazilian Journal of Medical and Biological Research. 2009;42:1080-5.

22. Neder, JÂ, Nery, LE. Clinical Exercise Physiology: Theory and Practice. Editora Artes Médicas. 2002.

23. Brazilian Society of Cardiology. II Guidelines on Exercise Testing. Arq Bras Cardiol. 2002;78(2).

24. Pollock, M, Franklin, BA, Balady, JG, Fletcher, B. Resistance exercise in individuals with and without cardiovascular disease. Circulation. 2000;101:828-33.

25. Neder, A, Nery, LE. Clinical Exercise Physiology: Theory and Practice. Editora Artes Médicas. 2003.

26. Cooper, BC. Exercise in chronic pulmonary disease: aerobic exercise prescription. Med Sci Sports Exerc. 2000;33:671-9.

27. Probst, VS, Troosters, T, Pitta, F, Decramer, M, Gosselink, R. Cardiopulmonary stress during exercise training in patients with COPD. Eur Respir J. 2006;27:1110-8.

28. Pereira, AM, Clara, H, Pereira, E, Simoes, S, Remédios, I, Cardoso, J, Brito, J, Cabri, J, Fernhall, B. Impact of combined physical exercise on the perception of health status of people with chronic obstructive pulmonary disease. Rev Port Pneumol. 2010;16:737-57.

29. Casaburi, R, Bhasin, S, Cosentino, L, Porszasz, J, Sonfay, A, Lewis, MI. Effects of testosterone and resistance training in men with chronic obstructive pulmonary disease. AM J Respir Crit Care Med. 2004;170:870-8.

30. Simpson, K, Killian, K, Mccartney, N, Jones, NL. Randomized controlled trial of weightlifting exercise in patients with chronic airflow limitation. Thorax. 1992;47:70-5

31. Cote, CG, Celli, BR. Pulmonary rehabilitation and the BODE index in COPD. Eur Respir J. 2005;26:630-6.

32. Maltais, F, Simard, AA, Simard, C, Jobin, J, Desgagnes, P, Lebranc, P. Oxidative capacity of the skeletal muscle and lactic acid kinetics during exercise in normal subjects and in patients with COPD. Am J Respir Crit Care Med. 1996;153:288-93.

33. Allaire, J, Maltais, F, Doyon, JF, Noel, M, Leblanc, P, Carrier, G, et al. Peripheral muscle endurance and the oxidative profile of the quadriceps in patients with COPD. Thorax. 2004;59:673-8.

34. Nasis, I.J et al. Effects of interval-load versus constant-load training on the BODE index in COPD patients. Respiratory Medicine. 2009;103:1392-8.

35. Puhan, MA, Mador, MJ, Held, U, Goldstein, R, Guyatt, GH, Schunemann, HJ. Interpretation of treatment changes in 6-minute walk distance in patients with COPD. Eur Respir J. 2008;32:637-43.

36. Dourado, VZ, Godoy, I. Muscle reconditioning in COPD: main interventions and new trends. Revista Brasileira de Medicina do Esporte. 2004;10(4).

37. Sala, E, Roca, J, Marrades, RM et al. Effects of endurance training on skeletal muscle bioenergetics in chronic obstructive pulmonary disease. Am J Respir Crit Care Med. 1999;159:1726-1734.

38. Casaburi, R. Skeletal muscle function in COPD. Chest. 2000;117.

39. Wenger, NK, Froelicher, ES, Smith, LK et al. Cardiac rehabilitation as secondary prevention clinical practice guideline. AHCPR. 1995;17.

LIST OF ANNEXES

FEDERAL UNIVERSITY OF SÃO CARLOS
CENTER OF BIOLOGICAL AND HEALTH SCIENCES
SPECIAL RESPIRATORY PHYSIOTHERAPY LABORATORY

ANNEX 1

Informed Consent Form

You are being invited to take part in the research project entitled **"COMBINED PHYSICAL training FOR ELDERLY PATIENTS WITH chronic obstructive PULMONARY DISEASE"**, proposed by physiotherapist Victor Fernando Couto, which will be carried out at the UFSCar Special Respiratory Physiotherapy Laboratory. You have been selected to take part in an assessment which will consist of an interview, cardiorespiratory and muscle assessment. One of the forms of assessment is the six-minute walk test, which will be carried out on a track 28 meters long and two meters wide, in order to assess your tolerance to exertion. This test will last six minutes, and before and after the test, blood pressure will be measured, the concentration of oxygen in the blood and heart rate will be observed non-invasively, and the level of shortness of breath and tiredness and/or pain in the legs will be questioned. During the test, these factors will also be observed, and if you experience intense shortness of breath and/or tiredness/pain in your legs or a higher than normal heart rate, the test will be stopped, avoiding any risk to your health.

Another form of assessment you will undergo is that of body composition, which is carried out using a bioelectrical impedance scale, where you will be instructed to fast for at least 4 hours to avoid any alterations. On the day of the assessment, you should wear light clothing and, if possible, remove any objects that could alter the values obtained on the scale. The scale will show muscle mass, body fat, metabolic age, body water, bone mass and body weight. The level of breathlessness during your activities of daily living will also be assessed by means of questionnaires, in which your participation is not obligatory.

If you agree to take part in this study, you will undergo one hour of physical training, including thirty minutes of aerobic exercise on an exercise bike. After this period, you will have a five-minute rest break. After this break, you will perform three sets of fifteen repetitions on a piece of equipment called a leg press, which aims to increase the strength of your lower limbs and give you greater independence to carry out activities of daily living. Throughout the training you will be monitored for blood pressure, blood oxygen concentration, heart rate and asked about shortness of breath and fatigue in the lower limbs.

In order to carry out a more complete assessment, you will have to present all the tests (clinical, laboratory, radiological and others) that you have carried out, as well as providing a history of family history and any other information requested for the smooth running of this treatment.

The information obtained in this study will be used for statistical or scientific purposes, always safeguarding your privacy (name, address and telephone number) and cannot be consulted by lay people without your written authorization. You should be aware that these procedures will not put your health or life at risk.

I am aware that I can withdraw from participating in the project at any time, with prior notice to the researcher and without any kind of burden to me and I agree to participate in this study of my own free will and I understand its relevance.

I undertake, to the best of my ability, to continue with the evaluations until they are completed, with the aim, in addition to the benefits they will bring, of collaborating in the good performance of the scientific work of those responsible for this project.

For questions regarding this study, please contact:

\-   Victor Fernando Couto

e-mail: **victorfcouto@yahoo.com.br**

Sao Carlos,   from   20

Volunteer's signature

ANNEX 2

EVALUATION FORM

Name:____

Date of birth: _________ // ___ Sex:______

Address: ____

Telephone: ____________________ Marital status: ____________

Medical_____________________________Diagnosis: ____________________

ANAMNESIS

QP:

HMP: ____

HMA: ____

Height:cm HR rest:bpm RR rest:rpm Spü^ rest:%

Weight:______ kgResting_____________ BP   :   mmHg

Breathing Type: CostalDiaphragmatic   Mixed   ApicalParadoxal

Chest type: NormalBarrelChestDug Other: _____________________________

Postural Assessment: ____

Cough: PresentAbsentDyspnea   : Present Absent

Secretion: Present   Absent

Pulmonary auscultation:____

MEDICINES USED

Name	Dosage	Frequency
	37	

ANNEX 3

ANALYSIS OF BODY COMPOSITION

Name:_______________________________________ Age: ___________ Height:______

Date:

Time of last meal: _______________________________

Evaluation schedule: _______________________________

<u>EVALUATION</u>

WEIGHT	% BODY FAT	% BODY WATER	MUSCLE MASS	IMB	METABOLIC AGE	BONE MASS

ANNEX 4

ESCALA MEDICAL RESEARCH COUNCIL

Name: ____

Date: _____ _____// ___

	DYSPNEA SCALE
Classification	**Features**
☐ Grade I	Shortness of breath occurs when you do intense physical activity (running, swimming, playing sports).
☐ Grade II	Shortness of breath occurs when you walk briskly on the flat or uphill.
☐ Grade III	He walks more slowly than people of the same age due to lack of air; or when he walks on the flat, he has to stop to breathe.
☐ Grade IV	After walking a few meters or a few minutes on the flat, they have to stop to breathe.
☐ Grade V	Shortness of breath prevents you from leaving the house or you feel short of breath when you change your clothes.

ANNEX 5

SIX-MINUTE WALK TEST

Name: _________________________________ Group: ______________ Date:___/___/_____

HR Submàx:bpmPAₜ: /   PAF: /   **Ambient Temperature:**

	SpO2	FCo	FCp	Dyspnea	MMII
Rest					
2'					
4'					
6'					
Rec 1'					
3'					
6'					

Distance traveled:

ANNEX 6

CYCLE ERGOMETER INCREMENTAL TEST

Name: ____ **Date:**___ / ___ / _____

Age:Sex:Height:Weight:Schedule:

Last meal:Bronchodilator schedule

FCmàx:FCsubmàx:FCachieved:(%màx)

Distance traveled:____

Test interrupted by: ____

	Load (W)	SpO2	FCp	FCo	FCmon	PA	Dyspnea	MMII
Rest								
1	15							
2	25							
3	35							
4	45							
5	55							
6	65							
7	76							
8	85							
9	95							
10	105							
11	115							
	Des. 15W							
Rec 1'								
Rec 3'								

Rec 6'								

ANNEX 7

1-REPETITION MAXIMUM TEST

Name:_________________________________ Group: _____________ Date:___/___/____

Submaximal HR:bpm

LEG PRESS	SpO2	Fco	FCp	PA	EB - dyspnea	EB - lower limb pain
Rest						
Load ( )						
Break 2'						
Load ( )						
Break 2'						
Load ( )						
Break 2'						
Load ( )						
Break 2'						
Load ( )						
Break 2'						
Load ( )						
Break 2'						
Load ( )						
Break 2'						
Load ( )						
Break 2'						
Load ( )						
Break 2'						

ANNEX 8

COMBINED PHYSICAL TRAINING FORM

Name:FCsubmàx: ____ **bpm**

	SpO2 (%)	HR (bpm)	BP (mmHg)	Dyspnea	LOWER LIMBS
Home					
Final					

CYCLERGOMETER　　　DISTANCE TRAVELED:

Time (min)	Load (W)	SpO2 (%)	HR (bpm)	BP (mmHg)	Borg (Disp/MMII)
2					
4					
6					
8					
10					
12					
14					
16					
18					
20					
22					
24					
26					
28					
30					
	SpO2(%)	HR (bpm)	BP (mmHg)	Borg (Dyspnea)	Borg (lower limbs)

After 5 minutes					

LEG PRESS

45

Series	Load (Kg)	SpO2 (%)	HR (bpm)	BP (mmHg)	Borg (Disp/MMII)
1					
Rec. (2')					
2					
Rec. (2')					
3					

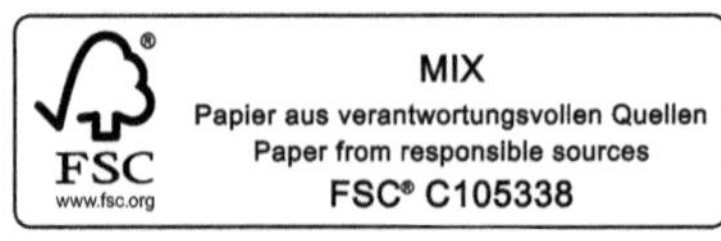

Printed by Books on Demand GmbH, Norderstedt / Germany